Immune Enhancing

Food Recipes To Quickly Boost And Enhance Your Immune System

By

John M. Crooks

© **Copyright 2021 by John M. Crooks- All rights reserved.**

This document is geared towards providing exact and reliable information in regards to the topic and issue covered. The publication is sold with the idea that the publisher is not required to render accounting, officially permitted, or otherwise, qualified services. If advice is necessary, legal or professional, a practiced individual in the profession should be ordered.

- From a Declaration of Principles which was accepted and approved equally by a Committee of the American Bar Association and a Committee of Publishers and Associations.

In no way is it legal to reproduce, duplicate, or transmit any part of this document in either electronic means or in printed format. Recording of this publication is strictly prohibited and any storage of this document is not allowed unless with written permission from the publisher. All rights reserved.

The information provided herein is stated to be truthful and consistent, in that any liability, in terms of inattention or otherwise, by any usage or abuse of any policies, processes, or directions contained within is the solitary and utter responsibility of the recipient reader. Under no circumstances will any legal responsibility or blame be held against the publisher for any reparation, damages, or monetary loss due to the information herein, either directly or indirectly.

Respective authors own all copyrights not held by the publisher.

The information herein is offered for informational purposes solely, and is universal as so. The presentation of the information is without contract or any type of guarantee assurance.

The trademarks that are used are without any consent, and the publication of the trademark is without permission or backing by the trademark owner. All trademarks and brands within this book are for clarifying purposes only and are the owned by the owners themselves, not affiliated with this document.

Table of contents

CHAPTER 1: ENTRÉE RECIPES 5

CHAPTER 2: SIDE DISH RECIPES 22

CHAPTER 3: SNACK RECIPES 31

CHAPTER 4: DESSERT RECIPES 38

Chapter 1: Entrée Recipes

1. Baked Salmon on a Bed of Cabbage, Fennel, and Apple

Yield: 4 plates

Servings: 4

Total Time: 40 minutes

Ingredients:

4 salmon filets

8 tablespoons olive oil

1/2 head of cabbage, chopped into small pieces 1 head of fennel, diced (or use 1 celery heart) 2 apples, peeled and diced

1/2 cup chicken broth (or water) 4 tablespoons of coconut oil

3-4 slices of bacon, chopped into pieces (optional) Salt and pepper, to taste

Directions:

1. Preheat oven to 350F.

2. Place each salmon filet onto a piece of aluminum foil with 2 tablespoons of olive oil and a bit of salt and pepper. Wrap up the aluminum foils and place in the oven for 30 minutes.

3. While the salmon is baking, place the coconut oil into a large saucepan and add in the cabbage and chicken broth and put the lid on the saucepan. After 10 minutes, add in the fennel, stir and keep the lid on. After another 10 minutes, add in the apples. Stir and season with salt and pepper. Cook until the salmon is done.

4. Place the cabbage mixture on a plate, place the salmon on top, then top with bacon pieces.

2. Cauliflower Crusted Pizza topped with Spinach and Prosciutto

Yield: 6 pizzas

Servings: 2

Total Time: 35 minutes

Ingredients:

1/2 head cauliflower

8 tablespoons olive oil

1 tablespoon garlic powder

1 tablespoon Italian seasoning

1/2 teaspoon salt

4 handfuls of spinach leaves

12 slices of prosciutto or ham (make sure there are no AIP-forbidden ingredients in the meat – check when you purchase it or alternatively top with chicken or other meat)

olive oil for greasing

Directions:

1. Preheat oven to 350F. Line a baking tray with parchment paper and then grease it with some olive oil.

2. Break the cauliflower into pieces, and food process the cauliflower with the 8 tablespoons olive oil, garlic powder, Italian season, and salt until it forms a soft mash.

3. Squeeze the water out of the cauliflower mash. Then divide into six.

4. Press each into a small pizza dough and bake in the oven for 20 minutes

until the crust turns slightly brown and harder.

5. While the crust is baking, boil a pot of water and drop the spinach into the boiling water. Boil for 1 minute and remove the spinach.

6. Place 2 slices of prosciutto onto each pizza (to prevent the spinach from making it soggy) then place the spinach on top.

7. Eat off the parchment paper as the crust is too fragile to remove.

3. Thai Chicken and Cauliflower Rice

Yield: 4 bowls

Servings: 4

Total Time: 30 minutes

Ingredients:

1 head of cauliflower

1 tablespoon freshly grated ginger 3 cloves of garlic, crushed

meat from a whole chicken (or use 3-4 cooked chicken breasts), shredded (you can use the chicken meat from the Slow Cooker Thai Chicken Soup) salt to taste

coconut oil to cook with

1 tablespoon coconut aminos (optional) 1/2 cup cilantro, chopped (for garnish)

Directions:

1. Break the cauliflower into florets and food process until it forms a rice-like texture (may need to be done in batches).

2. Place the cauliflower into a large pan with coconut oil and cook the cauliflower rice (may need to be done in 2 pans or in batches). Keep the heat on medium and stir regularly.

3. Add in the ginger and garlic.

4. When the cauliflower rice is soft, add in the shredded chicken meat.

5. Add in the coconut aminos and salt to taste. Mix well.

6. Garnish with cilantro.

7. Best served with a bowl of slow cooker Thai chicken soup.

4. Braised Cardamom Cabbage and Pork

Yield: 4 bowls

Servings: 4

Total Time: 2 hours 15 minutes

Ingredients:

1 lb pork (tenderloin or other cut), diced 1 head of cabbage, sliced

1 leek, sliced (or use an onion)

1 apple, peeled, cored, and diced

1 cup (16oz or 500ml) chicken broth (or water)

1/2 tablespoon cardamom powder 1 teaspoon turmeric

salt to taste

coconut oil to cook with

Directions:

1. Place 2 tablespoons of coconut oil into a large saucepan on high heat. When the oil is hot, add in the diced pork and sear the pork.

2. When all the pork pieces are browned, add in the chicken stock, cabbage, leek, apple, and spices.

3. Place the lid on the saucepan and simmer for 1 hour 30 minutes. Stir occasionally to ensure nothing sticks to the bottom of the saucepan.

4. It's done when the pork is tender (comes apart easily). Add salt to taste and serve.

5. Saffron Orange Acorn Squash Mash with Bacon and Collard Greens

Yield: 4 bowls

Servings: 4

Total Time: 1 hour

Ingredients:

1 lb bacon, diced

10 oz collard greens (approx. 1 bunch)

2 medium-sized acorn squash (or 1 butternut squash)

1/2 navel orange, finely chopped

pinch of saffron (crush and soak for 30 minutes in warm water)

Directions:

1. Preheat the oven to 400F.

2. Halve the acorn squash and remove the seeds. Then soften the inside of the squash by baking on a baking tray in the oven for 40 minutes at 400F (200C) or microwave on high for 3 minutes.

3. Cook the bacon in a pot until crispy.

4. Boil the collard greens in a pot of boiling water for 40 minutes until tender.

5. Scoop out the inside of the acorn squash when it's tender. Place the soft scooped-out acorn squash flesh into the pot with the beef bacon and the collard greens.

6. Add the orange and saffron (optional) to the pot and cook on a low heat

until the acorn squash forms a mash consistency (5-10 minutes).

7. Divide the "mash" into four bowls to serve.

6. Grilled Chicken Drumsticks with Garlic Marinade

Yield: 10 drumsticks

Servings: 2

Total Time: 30 minutes

Ingredients:

10 chicken drumsticks 1/2 cups of olive oil

1 head of garlic (around 10 cloves) juice from 1 lemon

1 tablespoon of sea salt

1/2 teaspoon of pepper

Directions:

1. Place the olive oil, garlic, lemon juice, sea salt, and pepper into a blender or food processor and puree. This is the marinade.

2. Rub the chicken drumsticks in the marinade.

3. Grill the chicken drumsticks.

7. Pan-Fried Pork Tenderloin with Peach and Basil Sauce

Yield: 2 plates

Servings: 2

Total Time: 30 minutes

Ingredients:

1 lb pork tenderloin salt and pepper to taste

1   tablespoon coconut oil

2   peaches, peel and chop into pieces 4 basil leaves

2 tablespoons coconut oil

1   teaspoon raw honey (optional)

Directions:

1.   Cut the 1 lb pork tenderloin in half (to create two equal shorter halves).

2.   Place the 1 tablespoon of coconut oil into a frying pan on a medium heat and fry the two pork tenderloin pieces in the pan.

3.   Leave the pork to cook on one side. Once that side is cooked, turn using tongs to cook the other sides. Keep turning and cooking until the pork looks cooked on all sides.

4.   Cook all sides of the pork until the meat thermometer shows an internal temperature of just below 145F (63C). The pork will keep on cooking a bit after you take it out of the pan.

5. While the pork is cooking, puree the peach pieces, basil leaves, 2 tablespoons of coconut oil, and the raw honey.

6. Let the pork sit for a few minutes and then slice into 1-inch thick slices with a sharp knife. Serve with the peach and basil sauce.

8. Pan-Fried Tilapia with Coconut Carrot Mash and Garlic Zucchini Sauté

Yield: 2 plates

Servings: 2

Total Time: 30 minutes

Ingredients:

2   tilapia filets

2 tablespoons coconut oil for frying 2 cups carrots, peeled and shredded 2 tablespoons coconut milk

1   zucchini, thinly sliced 3 cloves garlic, minced Salt to taste

Olive oil for frying

Directions:

1. Boil the carrots in a pot of water until tender (drain and puree). Mix with the coconut milk.

2. Sauté the zucchini with the garlic and olive oil. Salt to taste.

3. Pan-fry the tilapia in coconut oil – let it cook until most of the fish has turned from opaque to white.

4. Using a large spatula, turn the filets over and let it cook for a few more minutes.

5. Add salt to taste.

9. Pineapple Pork with Garlic and Cilantro

Yield: 2 bowls

Servings: 2

Total Time: 15 minutes

Ingredients:

2   cups of pineapple chunks (frozen or fresh)

3   cups of cooked shredded pork (or chicken) (pork or chicken made in advance in a slow cooker)

1 teaspoon freshly grated ginger 3 cloves of garlic, minced

1/4 cup of cilantro, chopped Salt and pepper to taste Coconut oil to cook in

Directions:

1.   Melt 1 tablespoon of coconut oil in a saucepan and add in the pineapple chunks.

2.   Drop in the shredded pork and cook for 5 minutes.

3.   Add in the ginger, garlic, cilantro, and season with salt and pepper to taste.

10. Slow Cooker Bacon and Chicken

Yield: 4 plates

Servings: 4

Total Time: 8 hours 5 minutes

Ingredients:

5 chicken breasts

10 slices of bacon (uncooked), chopped into small pieces 2 tablespoons thyme (dried)

1 tablespoon oregano (dried)

1 tablespoon rosemary (dried) (or use Italian seasoning instead of separate herbs)

5 tablespoons olive oil (2 tablespoons for the slow cooker and 3 tablespoons after cooking)

Directions:

1. Place everything into slow cooker, mix together, and cook for 8 hours on the low temperature setting.

2. Shred the meat and mix with 3 tablespoons of olive oil.

11. Slow Cooker Hearty Beef Stew

Yield: 4-6 bowls

Servings: 4

Total Time: 8 hours 20 minutes

Ingredients:

2 lbs beef (stew meat or short ribs meat), cubed 4 carrots, chopped

2 white parsnips, chopped 2 sweet potatoes, chopped 1 small onion, chopped

4 celery sticks, chopped 2 cloves of garlic, minced

1 14.5oz can of broth (beef, chicken, or vegetable or use water) 2 teaspoons of salt

1/2 teaspoon of black pepper

Directions:

1. Place everything into slow cooker, mix together, and cook for 8 hours on low temperature setting.

Chapter 2: Side Dish Recipes

12. Coconut Mashed Sweet Potatoes with Shredded Coconut and Ginger

Yield: large bowl

Servings: 4

Total Time: 35 minutes

Ingredients:

4 sweet potatoes

1   cup coconut milk 1 teaspoon of ginger

2   tablespoons shredded coconut (for topping)

Directions:

1. Bake the sweet potatoes at 350F (usually for over an hour) or boil or steam the sweet potatoes (usually for around 30 minutes). Make sure they are very tender - you should be able to poke a fork into them with ease.

2. Let the sweet potatoes cool for a bit and then peel them.

3. Place the peeled sweet potatoes into a food processor with the coconut milk and ginger, and food process on high until smooth.

13. Baked Parsnip Fries with Parsley

Yield: 1 large bowl

Servings: 4

Total Time: 50 minutes

Ingredients:

4 parsnips, peeled and cut into fries

1/4 cup parsley, finely chopped

1/4 cup olive oil 1 tablespoon salt

1 teaspoon black pepper

Directions:

1. Preheat oven to 450F.

2. Toss all the ingredients together in a large bowl and spread the fries onto a baking tray.

3. Bake for 40 minutes (move the fries around after 20 minutes to ensure they don't burn).

14. Lemon Asparagus Sauté with Bacon Topping

Yield: 1 large bowl

Servings: 2-4

Total Time: 20 minutes

Ingredients:

20 stalks of asparagus (approx.), chop off the end of the stalks and chop into small chunks

1   lemon

1/2 cup bacon bits/pieces, precooked salt to taste

Olive oil or bacon fat to cook with

Directions:

1. Sauté the asparagus in 2 tablespoons of olive oil.

2.   When the asparagus slices are tender, squeeze in the juice from 1 lemon (taste after squeezing in 1/2 a lemon to make sure how much more lemon juice you like).

3.   Add in the bacon bits and sauté for 2-3 minutes more.

4.   Add salt to taste.

15. Easy Bacon Brussels Sprouts

Yield: 1 very large bowl

Servings: 4-6

Total Time: 25 minutes

Ingredients:

2   lbs Brussels sprouts

1   lb bacon, uncooked (chopped into small pieces)

Directions:

1.   Chop off the ends from the Brussels sprouts and chop each in half.

2. Boil the halved Brussels sprouts for 10 minutes until tender.

3. While the Brussels sprouts are boiling, chop the bacon into small pieces (approx. 1/2-inch wide), and cook the bacon pieces in a separate large pot on

medium heat. When the bacon is crispy, add in the drained Brussels sprouts (so that the Brussels sprouts are in the pot with the bacon fat).

4. Cook for 10 more minutes, mixing occasionally to make sure nothing gets burnt on the bottom of the pan.

16. Roasted Turmeric Cauliflower

Yield: 1 large bowl

Servings: 4

Total Time: 1 hour 20 minutes

Ingredients:

Half of a large head of cauliflower 2 teaspoons of turmeric

2   teaspoons of salt

2 tablespoons of olive oil

Directions:

1.   Preheat oven to 350F (175C).

2.   Pull off florets from the cauliflower and combine with the turmeric, salt, and olive oil.

3.   Place in baking dish (spread out the cauliflower so they're not on top of each other), cover the baking dish with tin foil, and bake for 75 minutes.

17. Endives and Pear Sauté

Yield: 1 plate

Servings: 2

Total Time: 15 minutes

Ingredients:

4 endives, chopped into 1-inch chunks 1 pear, peeled and diced

2 cloves garlic, minced

1 teaspoon apple cider vinegar Salt to taste

Coconut oil to cook with

Directions:

1. Place 1 tablespoon of coconut oil into a frying pan on medium heat and add the endives.
2. When the endives start wilting a bit, add the minced garlic, diced pear, vinegar, and salt. Mix well.
3. Cook for 2 minutes and serve.

18. Ginger and Garlic Bok Choy Sauté

Yield: 1 plate

Servings: 2

Total Time: 15 minutes

Ingredients:

5 bok choy bunches

2 cloves of garlic, minced

1 teaspoon fresh ginger, grated salt to taste

coconut oil to cook in

Directions:

1. Cut off the ends of the bok choy. Then chop the bok choy into 1-inch long chunks.

2. Add 1 tablespoon of coconut oil into a saucepan (or wok) on a medium heat, and then add in the bok choy chunks. Stir frequently while the bok choy cooks.

3. After the bok choy starts to wilt, mix in the garlic, ginger, and salt to taste.

4. Cook for another 1-2 minutes and serve.

Chapter 3: Snack Recipes

19. Salt and Vinegar Kale Chips

Yield: 1 bowl

Servings: 1-2

Total Time: 20 minutes

Ingredients:

4 large kale leaves

1/2 tablespoon salt

2 tablespoons olive oil

1 teaspoon apple cider vinegar

Directions:

1. Wash the kale leaves and remove the stem so you're just left with leaves. Dry the leaves well.

2. In a bowl, add the leaves with the olive oil, salt and vinegar and mix well.

3. If using the oven, then preheat oven to 300F and place the leaves flat on a baking tray (with no overlapping). Bake for 5-10 minutes - make sure the leaves get crispy but not burned.

4. If using the dehydrator, then place the kale leaves flat on the dehydrator trays (with no overlapping) and dehydrate until crispy on 135F (3-5 hours).

5. If using a microwave, then place the kale leaves on a microwavable plate and place in microwave on full power for 2-3 minutes (check after 2 minutes to make sure they aren't burning).

20. Coconut Plantains Chips

Yield: 1 bowl

Servings: 2

Total Time: 45 minutes

Ingredients:

2   plantains, peeled and sliced really thin

approx. 1/2 cup coconut oil (depends how big the saucepan is)

salt to taste

Directions:

1. Place the coconut oil into a saucepan so that it's approx. 1/4 inch thick (or use a deep fat fryer to make this easier).

2. Heat up the oil for 3-4 minutes on a medium heat.

3. Drop in each thin slice of plantain one by one into the oil so they're not overlapping.

4. Use a perforated spoon to get the slices out as soon as they turn golden.

5. Repeat until all the slices are fried

6. Sprinkle with salt to taste.

21. Avocado Bacon Cups

Yield: 12 cups

Servings: 12

Total Time: 45 minutes

Ingredients:

30 thin slices of bacon

Equipment: standard nonstick metal muffin or cupcake pan 2 ripe avocados

Olive oil Balsamic vinegar Salt to taste

Directions:

1. Preheat oven to 400F.

2. Use 2 and 1/2 slices of bacon to make one bacon cup.

3. Turn the muffin cup over (the reverse side), and place 2 half slices of bacon across the back of one of the muffin cups. Place another half slice across those 2, perpendicular to those first 2 half slices. Then wrap a whole slice around the cup tightly.

4. Repeat for the other cups.

5. Bake for 25 minutes until crispy (place a baking tray underneath in the oven to catch any dripping bacon fat).

6. Cool for 5-10 minutes and then carefully remove the bacon cups from the back of the muffin tray. Store in the fridge until you're ready to enjoy (up to

a week).

7. Make the avocado filling when you're ready to eat: dice the avocado and toss with olive oil, balsamic vinegar, and salt to taste. Place into the bacon cups.

22. Baked Sweet Potato Chips

Yield: 1 large bowl

Servings: 4

Total Time: 40 minutes

Ingredients:

2 large sweet potatoes, peeled and thinly sliced 1 tablespoon coconut oil

1 teaspoon salt

Directions:

1. Preheat oven to 400F.

2. Toss the sweet potatoes with coconut oil and salt.

3. Spread in a single layer on 2 baking trays.

4.   Bake for 30 minutes (flip after 20 minutes).

5.   You'll need to watch them to make sure they don't burn. The exact time will depend on the thickness of the chips.

23.   Dehydrated Fruits and Vegetables

For vegetables (e.g., zucchinis), slice them into thin slices so it's faster to dry. Salting them (or dipping the slices into salt water) also makes them dry faster. For fruits, slice thin as well. Dehydration times using a dehydrator vary (longer from fruits generally). I suggest checking after 8-10 hours.

Chapter 4: Dessert Recipes

24. Pineapple Mango Banana Sorbet

Yield: 2 ramekins

Servings: 2

Total Time: 5 minutes

Ingredients:

1/2 cup frozen pineapples

1 cup frozen mango pieces 1 banana, room temperature

1/2 tablespoon fresh lime juice 1 banana for topping (optional)

Directions:

1. Place all the ingredients (except the banana for the topping) into a blender and blend really well. Depending on how good your blender is, you may have to blend briefly and then push the frozen fruit down and repeat several times.

2. Top with a few banana slices.

3.   Serve immediately.

25. Coconut Butter Stuffed Dates

Yield: 12 dates

Servings: 4

Total Time: 10 minutes

Ingredients:

12 pitted dates

1 cup coconut butter

Directions:

1.   Melt the coconut butter slightly in the microwave if it's not soft enough to scoop out with a spoon (make sure to take the metal lid off the jar first).

2.   Slice open each date so that it opens out but isn't sliced in half.

3.   Stuff each date with as much coconut butter as you can fit in while still being able to close it up.

26. Berry Jello

Yield: 2 cups

Servings: 2

Total Time: 4 hours

Ingredients:

1   cup of strawberries 1 cup of blueberries

2   tablespoons of gelatin powder 1 cup of water

1 teaspoon raw honey (optional)

Directions:

1.   Puree the strawberries and blueberries in a blender.

2.   Pour the pureed fruit into cups, filling each cup half way.

3.   Place 2 tablespoons of the gelatin powder into a large bowl and add in 1 cup of cold water. Stir well. Then place the bowl into the microwave and heat on high for 1 minute. Mix well using a fork.

4.   Pour the gelatin water into the cups with the fruit puree (almost filling each cup to the brim) and mix well.

5.   Leave in the fridge to set for 3-4 hours.

6.   Serve with a few slices of strawberries as garnish.

27. Vanilla Coconut Blueberry Bars

Yield: 8 bars

Servings: 4

Total Time: 1 hour 10 minutes

Ingredients:

1	cup coconut butter

2	tablespoons coconut oil 2 tablespoons raw honey 1 teaspoon vanilla extract 1/2 cup fresh blueberries 1/4 cup raisins (optional)

Directions:

1.	Gently melt the coconut butter, coconut oil, and honey. Add the vanilla extract.

2.	Line a 9 by 9 baking tray with parchment paper and pour the mixture in.

3.	Push the blueberries and raisins in and spread equally.

4.	Set in refrigerator for 1 hour.

5.	Cut into bars.

28. Strawberry Banana Macaroons

Yield: 12 macaroons

Servings: 4

Total Time: 1 hour 10 minutes

Ingredients:

2 fresh strawberries, chopped into 12 pieces 1 ripe banana

1 cup shredded coconut

1 teaspoon vanilla extract 2 tablespoons raw honey 2 tablespoons coconut oil

Directions:

1. Mash together the banana, coconut, vanilla, honey, and coconut oil.

2. Form into 12 balls.

3. Top each macaroon with a piece of strawberry.

4.	Refrigerate for 1 hour.

29. Microwave Banana Bread

Yield: 1 banana bread (approx. 1 cup)

Servings: 1

Total Time: 10 minutes

Ingredients:

1/4 cup coconut flour

2	1/2 tablespoons coconut oil, melted 1 ripe banana

1/2 teaspoon baking powder

1/2 teaspoon vanilla extract (optional)

Directions:

1.	Mix all the ingredients together in a microwaveable mug – mash the banana in with a fork.

2. Microwave on high for 90 to 120 seconds (1.5 to 2 minutes). Let the bread cool for a few minutes before eating from the mug (the bread is a bit crumbly).

30. 5-Minute Pumpkin Pie

Yield: 1 ramekin

Serves: 1

Total Time: 5 minutes

Ingredients:

6 tablespoons pumpkin puree 3 tablespoons coconut oil dash of cinnamon

dash of nutmeg dash of cloves

1 teaspoon raw honey

Directions:

1. Place all ingredients into a microwaveable bowl and microwave on high for approx. 45 seconds (just to make it easier to blend).

2. Blend well.

3. Serve immediately warm, or chill in refrigerator for a more solid consistency.

31. Cinnamon Pear and Butternut Squash Bowls

Yield: 4 bowls

Servings: 4

Total Time: 40 minutes

Ingredients:

1 butternut squash, chopped into 1/2 inch cubes 2 pears, peeled and chopped into 1/2 inch cubes 1 tablespoon raw honey

1 tablespoon cinnamon Coconut oil to cook with

Coconut cream to serve with (optional)

Directions:

1. Cook the butternut squash in 2-3 tablespoons of coconut oil in a large saucepan with the lid on for 10 minutes, stirring every few minutes.

2. Add in the pears, raw honey, and cinnamon.

3. Cook until the pears and the butternut squash are tender.

4. Divide into bowls and serve with coconut cream.

32. Apple Ginger Spice Sweet Potato Cookies

Yield: 10-15 cookies

Servings: 4

Total Time: 30 minutes

Ingredients:

1   medium sweet potato, cooked and mashed 1 apple, peeled

1/2 cup shredded coconut (optional) 1 teaspoon freshly grated ginger

2   tablespoons raw honey 1 teaspoon cinnamon

Directions:

1. Preheat oven to 350F and line a baking tray with parchment paper.

2. Blend or food process all the ingredients together.

3. Form small 2-inch diameter cookies (make them thin).

4. Bake for 20-25 minutes until they're pretty solid.

33. Raw Carrot Cake

Yield: 12 pieces

Servings: 4

Total Time: 2 hours 10 minutes

Ingredients:

1 cup carrots, finely chopped

1/2 cup shredded coconut

1 teaspoon freshly grated ginger

1/4 cup raw honey

1 tablespoon coconut oil 1 teaspoon vanilla extract 1 teaspoon lemon juice

1 teaspoon cinnamon 1/2 teaspoon nutmeg dash of cloves

Directions:

1. Press into a baking dish or just form using your hand into uniform 1-inch thick layer.
2. Refrigerate for 2-3 hours. Cut into squares or slices.